Leticia Calero

Psoriasis Diet Cookbook: Managing Symptoms with Delicious Anti-Inflammatory Recipes

This book was professionally typeset on Reedsy
Find out more at reedsy.com

Contents

    1.

    2.

    3.

    4.

    5.

    6.

    7.

    8.

    9.

1

Understanding Psoriasis and its Impact on Diet

<u>**I**ntroduction to Psoriasis:</u>

Psoriasis is a chronic autoimmune skin disorder that manifests as red, raised patches of skin covered with silvery-white scales. It is not a simple skin condition but rather a complex immune-mediated disorder. This condition occurs when the immune system mistakenly accelerates the skin's natural cycle of cell turnover, causing skin cells to accumulate rapidly on the surface. The result is the formation of distinct, often itchy, and sometimes painful patches of skin. These patches, known as plaques, can appear on various parts of the body, including elbows, knees, scalp, lower back, and even the face.

<u>**Characteristics of Psoriasis**</u>:

1. **Red and Inflamed Patches**: Psoriasis lesions are typically red, raised, and inflamed. The redness is caused by increased blood flow to the area due to inflammation, while the raised appearance is a result of the rapid accumulation of skin cells.

2. **Silvery-White Scales**: One of the hallmark features of psoriasis is the presence of silvery-white scales that cover the red patches. These scales are composed of dead skin cells and are a result of accelerated cell turnover.

3. **Itching and Discomfort**: Psoriasis patches are often itchy and can cause discomfort or even pain, especially if they crack or bleed. The urge to scratch can worsen the inflammation and potentially lead to further skin damage.

4. **Affected Areas:** Psoriasis can occur on any part of the body, but it commonly appears on areas with a higher density of sebaceous (oil) glands, such as the elbows, knees, and scalp. Additionally, it can affect nails, causing pitting, discolouration, and thickening.

5. **Chronic and Recurrent**: Psoriasis is a chronic condition, meaning it is long-lasting and can persist for years or even a lifetime. The symptoms can vary in severity over time, with periods of remis son (milder symptoms) and exacerbation (flare-ups).

6. **Triggers and Aggravators**: Various factors can trigger or worsen psoriasis flare-ups, including stress, infections, changes in weather, certain medications, and dietary choices. The link between diet and psoriasis severity is an area of ongoing research and is discussed in later chapters.

7. **Emotional Impact:** Beyond the physical symptoms, psoriasis can have a significant emotional and psychological impact. The visible

nature of the condition and potential social stigma can lead to feelings of self-consciousness, low self-esteem, and anxiety.

The connection between diet and psoriasis:

The connection between diet and psoriasis is an area of growing interest and research. While diet alone cannot cure psoriasis, it can play a significant role in managing its symptoms and improving overall well-being. Psoriasis is an autoimmune disorder characterized by the rapid buildup of skin cells, leading to the formation of inflamed, red, and often itchy patches on the skin. The severity and frequency of psoriasis flare-ups can be influenced by various factors, and diet is one of them.

Here's a deeper explanation of the connection between diet and psoriasis:

1. **Inflammation**: Psoriasis is associated with chronic inflammation in the body. Certain foods can either contribute to inflammation or help reduce it. A diet rich in processed foods, sugary snacks, and unhealthy fats can promote inflammation, potentially exacerbating psoriasis symptoms. On the other hand, a diet high in fruits, vegetables, whole grains, and healthy fats like those found in fish and nuts can have anti-inflammatory effects.

2. **Nutrient Intake:** Nutrient deficiencies have been linked to the development and progression of psoriasis. For example, deficiencies in vitamins D, A, and E, as well as omega-3 fatty acids, have been

observed in individuals with psoriasis. These nutrients play roles in immune function, skin health, and inflammation modulation. Including foods rich in these nutrients can positively impact psoriasis management.

3. **Gut Health**: Emerging research suggests a strong connection between gut health and psoriasis. The gut microbiome, the diverse community of microorganisms in the digestive tract, plays a crucial role in immune function and inflammation regulation. Specific diets, particularly those high in fibre and fermented foods, can promote a healthy gut microbiome, which in turn may help alleviate psoriasis symptoms.

4. **Trigger Foods:** Some individuals with psoriasis find that certain foods can trigger or worsen flare-ups. While trigger foods can vary from person to person, common culprits include alcohol, spicy foods, gluten, and dairy products. Identifying and avoiding trigger foods can lead to a reduction in symptom severity and frequency.

5. **Weight Management**: Obesity is associated with an increased risk of psoriasis and can worsen its symptoms. Maintaining a healthy weight through a balanced diet and regular exercise can help manage psoriasis and improve overall health.

6. **Stress Response**: Stress can trigger or exacerbate psoriasis flare-ups. Certain comfort foods that are high in sugar and unhealthy fats may be consumed during times of stress, potentially leading to inflammation and worsening of symptoms. Incorporating stress-

reducing foods like whole grains, leafy greens, and foods rich in antioxidants can be beneficial.

How inflammation and immune response play a role:

Inflammation and Immune Response in Psoriasis:

Psoriasis is fundamentally an autoimmune disorder, which means that the body's immune system mistakenly attacks healthy cells, in this case, skin cells. In individuals with psoriasis, this immune response is triggered by a complex interplay of genetic factors, environmental triggers, and immune system dysfunction.

Immune System Dysfunction:

In a healthy immune system, immune cells and molecules work together to protect the body from harmful invaders like bacteria and viruses. However, in people with psoriasis, specific immune cells, particularly T cells, become overactive. These T cells move to the skin and release inflammatory chemicals, such as cytokines, which are responsible for the redness, inflammation, and rapid growth of skin cells seen in psoriasis lesions.

Abnormal Proliferation of Skin Cells:

The immune system's hyperactivity in psoriasis leads to the rapid production of skin cells. Usually, skin cells take about a month to mature and move to the skin's surface. In psoriasis, this process is significantly sped up, taking just a few days. As a result, the excess skin cells accumulate on the skin's surface, forming the characteristic plaques or scales seen in psoriasis.

Role of Inflammation:

Inflammation is a natural response to injury or infection. However, in psoriasis, the immune system triggers inflammation even when there is no apparent threat. This persistent inflammation not only leads to the physical symptoms of redness, itching, and pain but can also contribute to the chronic nature of the disease.

Inflammatory Cytokines:

Cytokines are small proteins produced by immune cells that act as messengers to regulate immune responses. In psoriasis, specific cytokines, such as tumour necrosis factor-alpha (TNF-alpha) and interleukins, play a central role in promoting inflammation and the abnormal growth of skin cells. This cytokine imbalance contributes to the ongoing inflammation and the development of psoriatic lesions.

The Gut-Skin Connection:

Recent research has also highlighted the potential link between gut health and psoriasis. An unhealthy gut microbiome and increased intestinal permeability ("leaky gut") can lead to the release of pro-inflammatory substances into the bloodstream. These substances can potentially exacerbate inflammation and immune responses, further influencing the severity of psoriasis.

Diet's Influence on Inflammation and Immune Response:

Certain dietary factors can impact inflammation and immune response. Diets high in processed foods, sugary snacks, and unhealthy fats have been associated with increased inflammation. Conversely, diets rich in antioxidants, omega-3 fatty acids, and other nutrients can have anti-inflammatory effects. This is where diet comes into play in the management of psoriasis – by choosing foods that reduce inflammation, individuals may be able to mitigate the severity of their symptoms.

2

Breakfast Boosters

Recipe: Quinoa Breakfast Bowl with Fresh Berries

Quinoa, a versatile pseudo-grain, serves as the foundation for this breakfast, providing a combination of protein, fibre, and essential nutrients. The addition of fresh berries not only adds a burst of vibrant colour but also contributes antioxidants and vitamins that are beneficial for your skin health.

Ingredients:

- 1 cup cooked quinoa (prepared according to package instructions)

- Assorted fresh berries (e.g., strawberries, blueberries, raspberries, blackberries)

- 1/2 cup Greek yoghurt or dairy-free alternative (coconut yoghurt, almond yoghurt)

- 1-2 teaspoons honey or maple syrup (optional, for sweetness)

- Chopped nuts (such as almonds, walnuts) for added crunch and healthy fats

Instructions:

1. Prepare Quinoa:

- Start by cooking the quinoa according to the package instructions. Typically, you'll use a 1:2 quinoa-to-water ratio. Bring the water and quinoa to a boil, then reduce the heat, cover, and let it simmer for about 15 minutes until the water is absorbed and the quinoa is fluffy.

2. Assemble the Bowl:

- In a serving bowl, begin by placing the cooked quinoa as the base. You can let the quinoa cool slightly before assembling the bowl.

3. Add Fresh Berries:

- Wash and prepare the fresh berries of your choice. Strawberries, blueberries, raspberries, and blackberries all work wonderfully in this recipe. Arrange the berries on top of the quinoa, creating a colourful and visually appealing arrangement.

4. Top with Greek Yogurt:

- Place a dollop of Greek yoghurt or a dairy-free alternative on one side of the bowl. The creamy yoghurt adds a tangy contrast to the sweetness of the berries and the nutty flavour of quinoa.

5. **Drizzle with Sweetener**:

- If desired, drizzle a teaspoon or two of honey or maple syrup over the berries and yoghurt. This step is optional, as the natural sweetness of the berries might be sufficient for your taste.

6. **Sprinkle Chopped Nuts**:

- For a satisfying crunch and added healthy fats, sprinkle a handful of chopped nuts (such as almonds or walnuts) over the top of the bowl.

7. **Final Touches**:

- If you like, you can sprinkle a touch of cinnamon or a few mint leaves over the bowl for extra flavour and aroma.

8. **Serve and Enjoy**:

- Your Quinoa Breakfast Bowl with Fresh Berries is now ready to be enjoyed! Use a spoon to gently mix the components before each bite to combine all the flavours and textures.

Recipe: Avocado and Spinach Breakfast Smoothie:

Ingredients:

- 1 ripe avocado, peeled and pitted
- Handful of fresh spinach leaves
- 1 banana
- 1 cup almond milk (or any preferred milk)

- 1 tablespoon chia seeds or flax seeds (optional, for added fibre and omega-3 fatty acids)

- Ice cubes (as needed for desired thickness)

Method:

1. Prepare Ingredients: Begin by gathering all the necessary ingredients and preparing them for blending.

2. **Combine Avocado and Greens**: In a high-speed blender, add the ripe avocado (make sure it's soft and easy to blend) and the fresh spinach leaves. Avocado is rich in healthy monounsaturated fats, which can help support skin hydration and reduce inflammation. Spinach is loaded with vitamins A and C, both of which are beneficial for skin health.

3. **Add Banana for Creaminess**: Peel the banana and add it to the blender. Bananas not only add natural sweetness but also provide potassium and fibre.

4. **Pour in Almond Milk:** Pour in the almond milk or your preferred milk alternative. Almond milk is a great source of vitamin E and antioxidants, which can contribute to skin health.

5. **Include Seeds (Optional):** If desired, add chia seeds or flax seeds to the blender. These seeds are rich in fibre and omega-3 fatty acids, which can have anti-inflammatory benefits.

6. **Blend Until Smooth:** Start the blender on a low speed and gradually increase to high. Blend until all the ingredients are completely smooth and well combined. If the mixture is too thick, you can add a little more almond milk or water to reach your desired consistency.

7. **Adjust Thickness:** If you prefer a thicker smoothie, you can add a few ice cubes and blend again until they're fully incorporated.

8. **Serve and Enjoy:** Once the smoothie has reached your desired consistency, pour it into a glass. You can optionally garnish with a sprinkle of chia seeds, a slice of avocado, or a few spinach leaves. Sip and enjoy the refreshing and nutrient-packed smoothie.

<u>Recipe: Oatmeal with Almond Butter and Banana Slices:</u>

Ingredients:
- 1/2 cup rolled oats
- 1 cup water or milk of your choice (such as almond milk, oat milk, or dairy milk)
- 1 tablespoon almond butter
- 1 ripe banana, sliced
- 1/2 teaspoon cinnamon (optional)
- Chopped nuts (such as almonds, walnuts) for garnish (optional)
- Honey or maple syrup for sweetness (optional)

Method:

1. Prepare the Oatmeal:

- In a saucepan, combine the rolled oats and water or milk.

- Bring the mixture to a boil, then reduce the heat to a simmer.

- Stir occasionally and cook for about 5-7 minutes, or until the oats are soft and the mixture has thickened to your desired consistency.

2. Add Almond Butter:

- Once the oatmeal is cooked, remove the saucepan from the heat.

- Stir in the almond butter until it's well incorporated into the oatmeal. The almond butter will add a creamy texture and nutty flavour to the oatmeal.

3. Slice the Banana:

- Take a ripe banana and slice it into thin rounds. The banana adds natural sweetness, potassium, and additional texture to the oatmeal.

4. Assemble the Bowl:

- Transfer the almond butter-infused oatmeal to a serving bowl.

5. Add Banana and Flavor:

- Arrange the banana slices on top of the oatmeal. You can lay them out in a decorative pattern or simply scatter them over the surface.

- If desired, sprinkle cinnamon over the banana slices. Cinnamon adds a warm, comforting flavour and has potential anti-inflammatory properties.

6. Optional Garnishes:

- If you'd like, top the oatmeal with a handful of chopped nuts, such as almonds or walnuts. Nuts provide extra crunch, healthy fats, and additional nutrients.

7. Sweeten to Taste:

- If you prefer sweeter oatmeal, drizzle a small amount of honey or maple syrup over the top. Be mindful of the amount to keep the dish balanced and avoid excessive sugars.

8. Enjoy Your Oatmeal with Almond Butter and Banana:

- Grab a spoon and dig into your warm and comforting oatmeal bowl. The combination of creamy almond butter, sweet banana slices, and wholesome oats makes for a satisfying and nourishing breakfast.

3

Nourishing Lunches

Recipe 1: Grilled Chicken and Mixed Greens Salad with Turmeric Dressing

Ingredients:

- **Boneless, skinless chicken breast:** A lean source of protein that's essential for tissue repair and immune function.

- **Mixed greens (spinach, kale, arugula, etc.):** Packed with vitamins, minerals, and antioxidants that promote overall health.

- **Cherry tomatoes**: Provide a burst of flavour and are rich in vitamins A and C.

- **Bell peppers (assorted colours):** Vibrant and crunchy, these peppers offer a healthy dose of vitamin C.

- **Cucumber**: Hydrating and low-calorie, cucumbers add freshness and texture to the salad.

- **Red onion**: Adds a mild onion flavour and antioxidants.

- **Turmeric dressing:** Turmeric is known for its anti-inflammatory properties, and the dressing enhances both flavor and health benefits.

Preparation:

1. **Grill the Chicken:** Season the chicken breast with salt, pepper, and a touch of olive oil. Grill until cooked through, achieving a nicely charred exterior. Allow it to rest before slicing it into thin strips.

2. **Prepare the Grflavour**Wash and thoroughly dry the mixed greens. Tear or chop them into manageable pieces for easy eating.

3. **Chop the Vegetables**: Dice the cherry tomatoes, bell peppers, cucumber, and red onion. These colourful veggies will add both flavour and visual appeal to the salad.

4. **Make the Turmeric Dressing**: Create a turmeric dressing by mixing olive oil, lemon juice, ground turmeric, a pinch of black pepper (which enhances turmeric absorption), and a bit of honey or maple syrup for a touch of sweetness. Whisk until well combined.

Assembly:

1. **Assemble the Salad:** In a large bowl, combine the mixed greens, diced vegetables, and sliced grilled chicken.

2. **Drizzle with Dressing**: Drizzle the turmeric dressing over the salad. Toss gently to ensure an even distribution of flavours.

3. **Serve**: Portion the salad onto plates or bowls. Consider adding additional toppings like toasted nuts, seeds, or crumbled feta cheese for extra taste and texture.

Benefits:

- **Lean Protein:** The grilled chicken supplies high-quality protein, which is crucial for repairing and maintaining skin and other tissues.

- **Antioxidants:** The mix of colourful vegetables provides a range of antioxidants that help combat oxidative stress and inflammation.

- **Turmeric's Anti-Inflammatory Properties:** Turmeric contains curcumin, a compound known for its anti-inflammatory effects. Incorporating it into the dressing enhances the salad's potential to support psoriasis management.

Recipe 2: Lentil and Vegetable Stew

Ingredients:
- 1 cup dried green or brown lentils, rinsed and drained
- 1 onion, chopped
- 2 cloves garlic, minced
- 2 carrots, peeled and chopped
- 2 celery stalks, chopped
- 1 red bell pepper, chopped
- 1 zucchini, chopped
- 1 can (14 oz) diced tomatoes, with their juices
- 4 cups vegetable broth or water
- 1 teaspoon ground cumin
- 1 teaspoon ground coriander
- 1 bay leaf

- Salt and black pepper, to taste

- Fresh parsley or cilantro, chopped (for garnish)

Instructions:

1. **Sauté Aromatics**: In a large pot or Dutch oven, heat a tablespoon of olive oil over medium heat. Add the chopped onion and garlic, and sauté until the onion becomes translucent and fragrant.

2. **Add Vegetables**: Add the chopped carrots, celery, red bell pepper, and zucchini to the pot. Sauté for a few minutes until the vegetables begin to soften.

3. **Add Spices:** Sprinkle in the ground cumin and coriander. Stir to coat the vegetables with the spices, allowing the flavors to bloom.

4. **Lentils and Liquid**: Add the rinsed lentils, canned diced tomatoes (with juices), and vegetable broth (or water) to the pot. Stir everything together.

5. **Season and Simmer**: Drop in the bay leaf and season with salt and black pepper to taste. Bring the flavours to a boil, then reduce the heat to low, cover the pot, and let it simmer for about 25-30 minutes, or until the lentils are tender.

6. **Adjust Consistency:** If the stew becomes too thick as it simmers, you can add a bit more vegetable broth or water to achieve your desired consistency.

7. **Serve**: Once the lentils are cooked and the vegetables are tender, remove the bay leaf. Ladle the stew into bowls and garnish with chopped fresh parsley or cilantro.

Note:

- This lentil and vegetable stew is not only rich in plant-based protein and fibre but also provides an array of vitamins and minerals from the various vegetables.

- The combination of spices, including cumin and coriander, adds depth and warmth to the stew while also offering potential anti-inflammatory benefits.

- Feel free to customize the stew by adding other vegetables you enjoy or adjusting the seasoning to your taste.

- This stew can be prepared in larger batches and stored in the refrigerator or freezer for convenient, ready-to-heat lunches.

Recipe 3: Brown Rice Wrap with Hummus and Veggies

Ingredients:

- Brown rice tortillas (gluten-free alternative)
- Hummus (store-bought or homemade)
- Assorted vegetables (such as shredded carrots, bell peppers, cucumber, spinach, and any other preferred veggies)

- Optional additions: avocado slices, sprouts, microgreens, grilled tofu or chicken

Instructions:

1. **Prepare the Vegetables:**

Wash, peel, and chop the vegetables according to your preference. Aim for a variety of colours to ensure a range of nutrients and flavours.

2. **Warm the Tortillas:**

If the brown rice tortillas are too stiff, you can lightly warm them on a dry skillet or in the microwave. This makes them more pliable and easier to roll.

3. **Spread Hummus:**

Lay out a tortilla and spread a generous layer of hummus over the surface. Hummus not only adds creaminess but also provides plant-based protein and healthy fats.

4. **Layer the Vegetables:**

Arrange the chopped vegetables in a single layer over the hummus. Start with leafy greens like spinach, followed by shredded carrots, sliced bell peppers, cucumber, and any other veggies you choose.

5. Add Optional Ingredients:

If desired, include additional ingredients like avocado slices, sprouts, microgreens, or even some grilled tofu or chicken for extra protein and flavor.

6. Roll Up the Wrap:

Carefully fold in the sides of the tortilla and then roll it up from the bottom, keeping the fillings snug. The hummus will act as a glue to hold the wrap together.

7. Slice and Serve:

Once rolled, you can slice the wrap diagonally and favourite two halves, making it easier to eat. Serve the slices with your favourite side, such as a small salad or a handful of veggie chips.

4

Wholesome Dinners

Recipe: Baked Salmon with Roasted Brussels Sprouts

Ingredients:

- 2 salmon fillets

- 2 cups Brussels sprouts, trimmed and halved

- 2 tablespoons olive oil

- 1 lemon, juiced and zested

- 2 cloves garlic, minced

- 1 teaspoon fresh rosemary or thyme, chopped

- Salt and black pepper, to taste

Instructions:

1. Preheat the Oven:

- Preheat your oven to 400°F (200°C). Line a baking sheet with parchment paper or lightly grease it.

2. Prepare the Brussels Sprouts:

- Wash and trim the Brussels sprouts, removing any outer leaves that may be damaged. Cut them in half to ensure even roasting.

3. Toss Brussels Sprouts:

- In a mixing bowl, combine the halved Brussels sprouts with 1 tablespoon of olive oil, a pinch of salt, and a pinch of black pepper. Toss until the Brussels sprouts are well coated.

4. Arrange on the Baking Sheet:

- Spread the seasoned Brussels sprouts evenly on the prepared baking sheet, leaving space in the centre for the salmon fillets.

5. Prepare the Salmon:

- Place the salmon fillets on a plate. Drizzle the lemon juice and remaining olive oil over the fillets. Sprinkle with minced garlic, chopped rosemary or thyme, lemon zest, salt, and black pepper. Gently rub the seasonings into the fillets.

6. Place Salmon on Brussels Sprouts:

- Carefully place the seasoned salmon fillets in the centre of the baking sheet, over the bed of Brussels sprouts.

7. Bake:

- Transfer the baking sheet to the preheated oven and bake for about 15-20 minutes, or until the salmon is cooked to your desired level of doneness. The internal temperature of the salmon should reach 145°F (63°C).

8. **Check Brussels Sprouts:**

   - During baking, occasionally shake the baking sheet or gently toss the Brussels sprouts to ensure even roasting. They should be tender and slightly caramelized on the edges.

9. **Serve**:

   - Once the salmon and Brussels sprouts are cooked, remove the baking sheet from the oven. Carefully transfer the salmon fillets and Brussels sprouts to serving plates.

10. **Garnish and Enjoy:**

   - Garnish with additional fresh herbs, if desired. Serve the baked salmon with the roasted Brussels sprouts and any side dishes you prefer, such as quinoa, brown rice, or a mixed green salad.

Tips:

   - You can customize the seasoning for the salmon based on your preferences. Consider using other herbs like dill, thyme, or parsley.

   - If you prefer a bit of heat, you can add a pinch of red pepper flakes to the salmon seasoning.

   - Make sure to keep an eye on the salmon while baking to prevent overcooking, as the exact cooking time can vary based on the thickness of the fillets.

This delicious and nutritious recipe combines the omega-3-rich salmon with the health benefits of Brussels sprouts for a satisfying and psoriasis-friendly dinner option.

Recipe: Zucchini Noodles with Tomato and Basil Sauce

Ingredients:
- 3 medium zucchinis
- 4-5 ripe tomatoes, chopped
- 1/2 cup fresh basil leaves, chopped
- 3-4 cloves garlic, minced
- 2-3 tablespoons olive oil
- 1/4 teaspoon red pepper flakes (adjust to taste)
- Salt and black pepper to taste

Instructions:

1. **Prepare the Zucchini Noodles:**
    - Wash the zucchinis thoroughly and trim off the ends.
    - Use a spiralizer to create zucchini noodles. If you don't have a spiralizer, you can also use a julienne peeler to create thin strips resembling noodles. Place the zucchini noodles in a colander, sprinkle with a pinch of salt, and allow them to drain for about 15-20 minutes. This helps to remove excess moisture.

2. **Prepare the Tomato and Basil Sauce:**

- Heat a large pan over medium heat and add 2 tablespoons of olive oil.

- Add the minced garlic and red pepper flakes to the pan and sauté for about 1 minute until fragrant. Be careful not to burn the garlic.

- Add the chopped tomatoes to the pan and let them cook down, stirring occasionally. This should take about 10-15 minutes until the tomatoes break down and form a sauce.

- Once the tomatoes have cooked down, stir in half of the chopped basil leaves and season with salt and black pepper to taste. Allow the sauce to simmer for an additional 5 minutes to let the flavours meld.

3. **Cook the Zucchini Noodles**:

- While the sauce is simmering, gently pat the zucchini noodles dry with paper towels to remove excess moisture.

- Heat a separate pan over medium heat and add a tablespoon of olive oil.

- Add the zucchini noodles to the pan and sauté them for about 2-3 minutes until they are just slightly softened. Be careful not to overcook them; you want the noodles to maintain some crunch.

4. **Combine and Serve:**

- Add the sautéed zucchini noodles to the tomato and basil sauce, tossing them gently to coat with the sauce.

- Serve the zucchini noodles in individual bowls, topped with the remaining chopped basil leaves for a burst of fresh flavour.

- Optionally, you can garnish with a drizzle of extra virgin olive oil and a sprinkle of grated Parmesan cheese or nutritional yeast for added depth of flavour.

Notes:

- This recipe is naturally gluten-free and low in carbohydrates, making it suitable for those with dietary restrictions or seeking a lighter meal option.

- You can customize the level of spiciness by adjusting the amount of red pepper flakes used.

- Feel free to experiment with additional vegetables or protein sources to make the dish even more well-rounded.

Recipe: Tofu Stir-Fry with Broccoli and Bell Peppers

Ingredients:
- 1 block of firm tofu, pressed and cubed
- 2 cups broccoli florets
- 2 bell peppers (assorted colours), sliced
- 2 tablespoons tamari or soy sauce (low-sodium if preferred)
- 1 tablespoon fresh ginger, minced
- 2 cloves garlic, minced
- 1 tablespoon sesame oil
- 1 tablespoon sesame seeds
- Optional: Red pepper flakes for added heat
- Cooked rice or quinoa, for serving

Instructions:

1. **Prepare the Tofu:**

   - Start by pressing the tofu to remove excess moisture. Wrap the tofu block in a clean kitchen towel and place a heavy object (like a plate) on top. Let it sit for about 20-30 minutes. Then, cut the tofu into bite-sized cubes.

2. **Sauté Aromatics:**

   - In a large wok or skillet, heat the sesame oil over medium-high heat. Add the minced ginger and garlic. Sauté for about 1-2 minutes until fragrant.

3. **Cook the Tofu:**

   - Carefully add the cubed tofu to the wok. Spread the tofu evenly to allow it to brown. Let it cook undisturbed for a few minutes until the bottom side is golden brown. Then, gently toss the tofu to brown the other sides. This will take about 5-7 minutes.

4. **Add Vegetables:**

   - Add the broccoli florets and sliced bell peppers to the wok. Stir-fry for about 3-4 minutes until the vegetables start to soften but are still vibrant in colour. Adjust the heat as needed to prevent burning.

5. Flavor with Tamari:

- Drizzle the tamari or soy sauce over the tofu and vegetables. Toss everything together to ensure the flavours are well distributed. If you like a bit of heat, you can also add red pepper flakes at this stage.

6. Final Touch:

- Sprinkle the sesame seeds over the stir-fry and give it a final toss. The sesame seeds not only add a delightful crunch but also a nutty flavour that complements the dish perfectly.

7. Serve:

- Serve the tofu stir-fry over cooked rice or quinoa for a complete meal. The grains will soak up the delicious flavours of the stir-fry and provide a satisfying base.

5

Snacks and Appetizers for Psoriasis Relief

Recipe: Guacamole with Veggie Sticks

Guacamole is a beloved dip that's not only delicious but also offers a wealth of nutritional benefits. This recipe combines the creamy richness of avocados with the vibrant flavours of tomatoes, red onion, garlic, lime juice, and cilantro. Paired with an array of fresh veggie sticks, this guacamole becomes a wholesome and satisfying snack that's perfect for soothing psoriasis symptoms and supporting overall health.

Ingredients:
- 2 ripe avocados, peeled and pitted
- 1 small red onion, finely chopped
- 1-2 tomatoes, diced
- 1-2 cloves garlic, minced
- Juice of 1 lime
- Fresh cilantro, chopped

- Salt and pepper to taste

- Assorted veggie sticks (carrots, cucumber, bell peppers, etc.) for dipping

Instructions:

1. **Prepare the Avocados:**

- Cut the avocados in half lengthwise. Carefully remove the pits and scoop out the flesh into a mixing bowl.

2. **Mash the Avocados:**

- Use a fork to mash the avocado flesh until you achieve your desired level of smoothness. Some prefer a chunkier texture, while others enjoy a creamier consistency.

3. **Add the Flavors:**

- Add the finely chopped red onion to the mashed avocado. The red onion provides a mild bite and adds a pleasant crunch.

- Dice 1-2 tomatoes and add them to the mixture. Tomatoes not only bring vibrant colour but also a burst of juiciness and natural sweetness.

4. **Introduce Garlic and Lime:**

- Mince 1-2 cloves of garlic and incorporate them into the mixture. Garlic enhances the flavour profile and provides potential health benefits.

- Squeeze the juice of 1 lime into the bowl. Lime juice adds a refreshing citrusy tang and helps prevent the avocados from browning.

5. Enhance with Cilantro:

- Chop a handful of fresh cilantro leaves and add them to the mixture. Cilantro contributes a bright, herbaceous note that balances the richness of the avocado.

6. Season and Mix:

- Season the guacamole with salt and pepper to taste. Start with a small amount and adjust according to your preference.
- Gently mix all the ingredients, ensuring that the flavours are well combined.

7. Serve with Veggie Sticks:

- Wash and prepare an assortment of veggie sticks, such as carrot sticks, cucumber slices, and bell pepper strips.
- Arrange the veggie sticks on a serving platter alongside a bowl of freshly made guacamole.

8. Enjoy:

- Dip the veggie sticks into the guacamole and savour the vibrant combination of flavours, textures, and nutrients.

Note: Guacamole is best enjoyed immediately after preparation to retain its freshness and vibrant colour. If you need to store it for a short period, cover the bowl with plastic wrap, ensuring it directly touches the guacamole's surface to minimize oxidation.

Recipe: Roasted Chickpeas with Turmeric and Cumin

Ingredients:
   - 1 can (15 oz) chickpeas, drained and rinsed
   - 1 tablespoon olive oil
   - 1 teaspoon ground turmeric
   - 1/2 teaspoon ground cumin
   - 1/4 teaspoon ground coriander (optional, for extra flavour)
   - 1/4 teaspoon cayenne pepper (adjust to taste)
   - Salt to taste

Instructions:

1. **Preheat the Oven:**

Preheat your oven to 400°F (200°C). Preheating is important to ensure that the chickpeas roast evenly and become crispy.

2. **Prepare the Chickpeas:**

Drain and rinse the canned chickpeas thoroughly. Pat them dry using a clean kitchen towel or paper towel. Removing excess moisture helps achieve a crispy texture.

3. **Season the Chickpeas:**

In a mixing bowl, combine the dried chickpeas with olive oil, ground turmeric, ground cumin, ground coriander (if using), cayenne pepper, and a pinch of salt. Toss the chickpeas until they are evenly coated with the seasoning mixture. The turmeric and cumin not only add flavour but also provide anti-inflammatory benefits.

4. **Spread on Baking Sheet:**

Spread the seasoned chickpeas in a single layer on a baking sheet. This ensures that they roast evenly and become crunchy. You can line the baking sheet with parchment paper or lightly grease it to prevent sticking.

5. **Roasting Process:**

Place the baking sheet in the preheated oven and roast the chickpeas for about 20-25 minutes. It's a good idea to shake the baking sheet gently halfway through the roasting time to ensure even cooking. The chickpeas will start to turn golden and become crisp as they roast.

6. **Check for Crispiness:**

After the initial roasting time, check the chickpeas for crispiness. You can do this by taking one chickpea out and allowing it to cool for a moment. If it's not as crunchy as you'd like, put it back in the oven for a few more minutes.

7. **Cooling and Storage**:

Once the chickpeas are crispy to your liking, remove the baking sheet from the oven. Let the chickpeas cool on the baking sheet; they will continue to crisp up as they cool. Once completely cool, you can transfer them to an airtight container for storage.

8. **Enjoy Your Snack:**

Roasted chickpeas with turmeric and cumin make a fantastic snack that's not only satisfyingly crunchy but also packed with flavour and nutrition. Enjoy them on their own, toss them into salads for extra texture, or use them as a topping for soups.

Note: You can adjust the seasoning quantities according to your taste preferences. If you prefer a milder flavour, reduce the cayenne pepper or omit it altogether. Feel free to experiment with other spices like smoked paprika or garlic powder to create your own unique flavor profile.

Recipe: Greek Yogurt and Berry Parfait

Ingredients:

- 1 cup Greek yoghurt (plain or flavoured)
- 1/2 cup assorted berries (strawberries, blueberries, raspberries)
- 1 tablespoon honey or maple syrup (optional)
- 1/4 cup granola (optional)

Instructions:

1. **Prepare the Berries:**

- Wash the berries under cold water and pat them dry with a paper towel.

- If using strawberries, remove the stems and chop them into bite-sized pieces. Leave smaller berries like blueberries and raspberries whole.

2. **Assemble the Parfait:**

- Choose a glass, mason jar, or bowl for assembling your parfait.

- Start by spooning a layer of Greek yogurt into the bottom of the container.

3. **Layer the Berries:**

- Add a handful of the assorted berries on top of the yoghurt layer. You can use a mix of different berries for a burst of colours and flavours.

4. **Drizzle with Sweetener:**

- If you prefer a touch of sweetness, drizzle a teaspoon of honey or maple syrup over the berries. This adds a delightful contrast to the tangy yogurt and the natural sweetness of the berries.

5. **Repeat the Layers:**

- Create another layer by adding more Greek yogurt on top of the berries and sweetener.

6. Add Crunch with Granola:

- For an extra layer of texture, sprinkle a quarter cup of granola over the yogurt. The granola provides a satisfying crunch and complements the creaminess of the yogurt and the juiciness of the berries.

7. Final Touch:

- If you're using a clear glass or jar, the layers of yoghurt, berries, sweetener, and granola create a visually appealing presentation.

8. Serve and Enjoy:

- Your Greek Yogurt and Berry Parfait are ready to be enjoyed! You can eat it immediately or let it sit in the refrigerator for a little while to let the flavours meld together.

Variations:

- **Nutty Delight:** Add a sprinkle of chopped nuts (such as almonds, walnuts, or pecans) between the layers for an extra dose of healthy fats and crunch.

- **Chocolate Indulgence**: For a touch of indulgence, add a few chocolate chips or cocoa nibs between the layers.

- **Seeds and Superfoods**: Boost the nutritional value by adding chia seeds, flaxseeds, or acai berries to the layers.

6

Healing Beverages

Recipe: Anti-Inflammatory Turmeric Tea

Turmeric tea is a soothing and warming beverage that harnesses the anti-inflammatory properties of turmeric to provide potential relief for individuals with psoriasis. Turmeric contains an active compound called curcumin, which has been studied for its ability to reduce inflammation and oxidative stress in the body. This tea combines turmeric with other aromatic spices to create a flavorful and health-promoting drink.

Ingredients:

- 1 teaspoon ground turmeric
- 1/2 teaspoon ground ginger
- 1/4 teaspoon ground cinnamon
- 1 teaspoon honey (optional)
- 1 cup hot water
- Lemon wedge (for garnish)

Instructions:

1. **Prepare the Spices:**

In a mug, combine the ground turmeric, ground ginger, and ground cinnamon. These spices not only contribute to the tea's flavour but also provide potential anti-inflammatory benefits.

2. **Add Hot Water:**

Boil water and pour 1 cup of hot water into the mug with the spice mixture. Make sure the water is hot enough to steep the spices effectively.

3. **Stir and Dissolve:**

Use a spoon to stir the hot water and spices together. The spices should dissolve, creating a rich and fragrant mixture.

4. **Add Honey (Optional):**

If you prefer your tea slightly sweetened, add a teaspoon of honey to the mug. Honey not only adds sweetness but also contributes additional potential health benefits.

5. **Steep the Tea:**

Allow the tea to steep for a few minutes. During this time, the flavours from the spices will infuse into the water, creating a vibrant and aromatic blend.

6. **Garnish with Lemon:**

Squeeze a wedge of lemon into the tea. Lemon not only adds a refreshing tang but also provides a boost of vitamin C, which can support immune health.

7. **Stir and Enjoy:**

Stir the tea well to ensure that all the ingredients are mixed evenly. The warm and comforting aroma of the spices will entice your senses. Sip the tea slowly, savouring the flavours and potential benefits.

Note: If you're new to turmeric or have concerns about staining, you can use a small pinch of black pepper in the tea. Black pepper contains piperine, a compound that can enhance the absorption of curcumin from turmeric.

Recipe: Cucumber and Mint Infused Water

Ingredients:

- 1/2 cucumber, thinly sliced
- Handful of fresh mint leaves
- Ice cubes
- Water

Instructions:

1. **Prepare the Ingredients**:

- Wash the cucumber thoroughly under cold water.
- Thinly slice the cucumber into rounds. You can use a sharp knife or a mandoline slicer for even slices.

- Pick a handful of fresh mint leaves, gently rinsing them to remove any dirt or debris.

2. Assemble the Infusion:

- Choose a pitcher or a large glass container to hold the infused water.

- Place the cucumber slices at the bottom of the pitcher.

- Add the fresh mint leaves on top of the cucumber slices.

3. Add Ice Cubes:

- To keep the infused water cool and refreshing, add a generous amount of ice cubes to the pitcher. The ice will also help release the flavours from the ingredients.

4. Pour Water:

- Carefully pour cold water into the pitcher, covering the cucumber and mint. Use filtered or bottled water for the best taste.

5. Infuse the Water:

- Gently stir the ingredients with a long spoon to distribute the flavours.

- Let the water infuse for at least 30 minutes to an hour. You can even refrigerate the pitcher overnight for a stronger infusion.

6. Serve and Enjoy:

- Once the water is infused to your liking, it's ready to be enjoyed.

- To serve, you can use a ladle or a slotted spoon to scoop out cucumber slices and mint leaves along with the infused water.

- Pour the infused water into glasses, making sure to include a few cucumber slices and mint leaves in each glass for an appealing presentation.

Tips:

- Feel free to customize the flavours by adding other ingredients such as lemon slices, lime wedges, or berries.

- You can refill the pitcher with water a couple of times before the flavours start to weaken.

- For a more intense flavour, gently crush the mint leaves before adding them to the pitcher.

- If you prefer a slightly sweeter infusion, add a few slices of fresh fruit like strawberries or oranges.

Benefits:

- Cucumber is hydrating and contains vitamins and minerals that can support skin health.

- Mint provides a refreshing flavour and may have soothing properties for the digestive system.

- Drinking infused water encourages increased water intake, promoting hydration that is essential for managing psoriasis and overall well-being.

Recipe: Green Smoothie with Kale and Pineapple

Ingredients:

- 1 cup kale leaves, stems removed

- 1/2 cup fresh pineapple chunks

- 1/2 banana

- 1/2 cup coconut water

- 1/2 cup almond milk (or any preferred milk)

- 1 tablespoon chia seeds

- Ice cubes

Instructions:

1. **Prepare Your Ingredients:**
   - Wash the kale leaves thoroughly, and remove the tough stems.
   - Cut the pineapple into small chunks.
   - Peel and slice the banana.

2. **Assemble Your Blender:**
   - Place the kale leaves, pineapple chunks, banana slices, and chia seeds in a blender.

3. **Add Liquid Ingredients:**
   - Pour in the coconut water and almond milk. Coconut water provides natural sweetness and hydration, while almond milk adds creaminess.

4. **Add Ice Cubes:**
   - If you prefer a chilled smoothie, toss in a few ice cubes. This will also help achieve a refreshing texture.

5. Blend Until Smooth:

- Start blending at a low speed and gradually increase to high. Blend until all the ingredients are well combined and the smoothie reaches a smooth consistency.

6. Adjust Consistency:

- If the smoothie is too thick, you can add a bit more coconut water or almond milk and blend again until you achieve your desired thickness.

7. Taste and Adjust:

- Taste the smoothie and adjust sweetness by adding more pineapple or banana if needed. If you prefer a tangier flavour, you can also add a splash of fresh lemon juice.

8. Serve and Enjoy:

- Pour the smoothie into a glass.

- If you'd like, you can sprinkle a few chia seeds on top for added texture and nutrition.

- Insert a colourful straw and sip your delicious and nutrient-packed green smoothie.

Additional Tips:

- To make the smoothie even creamier, you can add a tablespoon of Greek yoghurt or a small scoop of plant-based protein powder.

- If you're not a fan of coconut water, you can substitute it with regular water or more almond milk.

- Feel free to customize the ingredients based on your preferences and dietary restrictions. You can replace kale with spinach, switch up the fruits, or add a touch of natural sweeteners like honey or maple syrup if desired.

Benefits of the Green Smoothie:

- **Nutrient-Rich:** This smoothie is packed with vitamins, minerals, and antioxidants from kale, pineapple, and banana. These nutrients can contribute to skin health and overall well-being.

- **Hydration**: The combination of coconut water and almond milk helps keep you hydrated, which is essential for managing psoriasis symptoms.

- **Digestive Support:** Chia seeds are a great source of dietary fibre, which aids digestion and promotes gut health.

- **Anti-Inflammatory:** Kale contains compounds that have been associated with anti-inflammatory properties, which may benefit individuals with psoriasis.

7

Psoriasis-Soothing Desserts

Chia Seed Pudding with Mixed Berries

Ingredients:

- 1/4 cup chia seeds

- 1 cup almond milk (or any preferred milk)

- 1 tablespoon honey or maple syrup (optional, for sweetness)

- 1 teaspoon vanilla extract

- Mixed berries (such as strawberries, blueberries, and raspberries)

Instructions:

1. **Prepare the Chia Seed Base**:

- In a bowl, combine the chia seeds, almond milk, honey or maple syrup (if using), and vanilla extract.

- Mix the ingredients well using a spoon or whisk. Make sure the chia seeds are evenly distributed and not clumped together.

2. **Allow the Mixture to Thicken**:

- Cover the bowl with plastic wrap or a lid.

- Place the bowl in the refrigerator and let it sit for at least 2 hours or overnight. During this time, the chia seeds will absorb the liquid and create a pudding-like consistency.

3. Stir and Check the Consistency:

- After the initial setting time, give the mixture a good stir. You'll notice that the chia seeds have expanded and created a thick, pudding-like texture.

- If the pudding seems too thick, you can add a little more almond milk to achieve your desired consistency.

4. Serve with Mixed Berries:

- Wash and prepare the mixed berries. You can slice strawberries, rinse blueberries and raspberries, or use any other berries you prefer.

- When you're ready to serve, divide the chia seed pudding into individual serving bowls or glasses.

5. Top with Mixed Berries:

- Generously layer the top of each serving with a variety of mixed berries.

- The vibrant colours and fresh flavours of the berries will not only enhance the visual appeal of the dish but also add extra antioxidants and vitamins.

6. Enjoy:

- Dig in and savour the creamy texture of the chia seed pudding combined with the burst of juiciness from the mixed berries.

- Feel free to get creative with additional toppings such as chopped nuts, coconut flakes, or a drizzle of more honey for added sweetness.

Tips:

- You can adjust the sweetness of the pudding by adding more or less honey or maple syrup according to your taste preferences.

- Experiment with different types of milk, such as coconut milk or oat milk, for varying flavours.

- For a smoother pudding texture, you can blend the chia seed mixture briefly before refrigerating it.

- Prepare a larger batch of chia seed pudding and store it in the refrigerator for quick and healthy snacks throughout the week.

Baked Apples with Cinnamon and Walnuts:

Ingredients:

- Apples (1 apple per serving, choose firm varieties like Granny Smith, Honeycrisp, or Fuji)
- Ground cinnamon
- Chopped walnuts
- Honey or maple syrup (optional)

Instructions:

1. **Preheat the Oven:** Preheat your oven to 350°F (175°C) to ensure it's ready for baking the apples.

2. **Prepare the Apples**: Wash and dry the apples thoroughly. Using an apple corer or a paring knife, carefully core the apples, removing the seeds and creating a well in the centre for the filling. Be sure not to cut through the bottom of the apple.

3. **Infuse with Cinnamon**: Sprinkle a generous pinch of ground cinnamon inside each cored apple, distributing it evenly around the inner surface and inside the well you've created.

4. **Add the Nutty Crunch**: Fill the wells of the apples with chopped walnuts. The walnuts will provide a delightful crunch and complement the soft texture of the baked apples.

5. **Sweeten if Desired:** Drizzle a small amount of honey or maple syrup into each apple well. This step is optional and can be adjusted based on your preference for sweetness.

6. **Bake the Apples:** Place the prepared apples in a baking dish or on a baking sheet, ensuring they are stable and won't tip over during baking. If desired, you can also place a small pat of butter on top of each apple to enhance the flavour and texture.

7. **Bake Until Tender**: Bake the apples in the preheated oven for about 20-25 minutes or until they are tender but still hold their

shape. The baking time may vary depending on the size and variety of apples you're using.

8. **Serve and Enjoy:** Once the apples are baked to perfection, carefully remove them from the oven and let them cool slightly before serving. The warmth of the baked apples combined with the aromatic cinnamon and the nutty walnuts creates a cosy dessert experience.

9. **Optional Garnish**: If you'd like to add a touch of elegance, consider garnishing the baked apples with a sprinkle of additional cinnamon or a drizzle of honey just before serving.

10. **Serve with Toppings:** Baked apples can be enjoyed on their own or served with a dollop of Greek yoghurt, a scoop of vanilla ice cream, or a drizzle of caramel sauce for an extra special treat.

Tip: For an extra burst of flavour, you can also experiment with adding dried fruits such as raisins or cranberries to the walnut filling.

Dark Chocolate Avocado Mousse:

Ingredients:
- 2 ripe avocados
- 1/4 cup unsweetened cocoa powder
- 1/4 cup honey or maple syrup (adjust to taste)
- 1 teaspoon vanilla extract

- A pinch of salt

- Dark chocolate shavings (for garnish)

Instructions:

1. **Prepare the Avocados:**

   - Cut the avocados in half and remove the pits.

   - Scoop out the flesh and place it in a food processor. Make sure the avocados are ripe for a smooth and creamy texture.

2. **Blend the Ingredients:**

   - Add the unsweetened cocoa powder, honey or maple syrup, vanilla extract, and a pinch of salt to the avocados in the food processor.

3. **Blend Until Smooth:**

   - Blend all the ingredients until you achieve a smooth and velvety consistency. Scrape down the sides of the processor as needed to ensure everything is evenly mixed.

4. **Taste and Adjust:**

   - Taste the mousse and adjust the sweetness by adding more honey or maple syrup if desired. Keep in mind that dark chocolate shavings will also contribute some sweetness.

5. **Chill the Mousse:**

- Transfer the mousse to individual serving cups or a larger bowl. Cover with plastic wrap, making sure the plastic touches the surface of the mousse to prevent oxidation.

- Refrigerate the mousse for about 1 hour to allow the flavours to meld and the mousse to firm up.

6. **Garnish and Serve:**

- Before serving, garnish the mousse with dark chocolate shavings. You can use a grater or a vegetable peeler to create the shavings.

7. **Enjoy**:

- Serve the Dark Chocolate Avocado Mousse chilled and savour the rich flavours and creamy texture. The mousse can be enjoyed on its own or paired with fresh berries, a dollop of whipped cream, or a sprinkle of chopped nuts.

8

Special Diets and Considerations

<u>**E**xploring **Gluten-Free, Dairy-Free, and Other Special Diets for Psoriasis Management:**</u>

Gluten-Free Diet:

A gluten-free diet involves avoiding foods that contain gluten, a protein found in wheat, barley, and rye. While not everyone with psoriasis needs to avoid gluten, some individuals may experience improvements in their symptoms by eliminating it from their diet. Gluten can trigger an immune response in certain individuals, leading to inflammation that may exacerbate psoriasis. This connection between gluten sensitivity and psoriasis is still being researched, but some individuals do report reduced symptoms when they follow a gluten-free diet.

Dairy-Free Diet:

Dairy products, such as milk, cheese, and yoghurt, are a common source of inflammation-triggering proteins and compounds. Some individuals with psoriasis find that their symptoms improve when they eliminate dairy from their diet. This could be due to lactose intolerance, casein sensitivity, or other components in dairy products that can contribute to inflammation.

Anti-Inflammatory Diet:

An anti-inflammatory diet focuses on consuming foods that are rich in antioxidants, omega-3 fatty acids, and other nutrients that can help reduce inflammation in the body. This type of diet can be beneficial for managing chronic inflammatory conditions like psoriasis. It emphasizes whole foods, such as fruits, vegetables, whole grains, lean proteins, and healthy fats.

Plant-Based Diet:

A plant-based diet emphasizes the consumption of foods derived from plants, including fruits, vegetables, whole grains, nuts, seeds, and legumes. Plant-based diets are often rich in antioxidants and other nutrients that can support overall health and potentially alleviate psoriasis symptoms.

<u>Tips for Navigating Social Situations and Dining Out While Adhering to Your Dietary Needs:</u>

1. **Communicating Your Needs:**

When attending social events or dining out, clear communication is key. If you have dietary restrictions due to psoriasis or other health reasons, it's important to let your hosts or the restaurant staff know about your requirements in advance. Politely explain your situation and ask if accommodations can be made. Most people and establishments are understanding and willing to work with you.

2. Planning Ahead:

Before attending an event or dining out, take some time to plan. If you're aware of the restaurant or menu in advance, review it online if possible. Look for dishes that align with your dietary needs. If you're unsure, consider contacting the restaurant to discuss your preferences and inquire about possible modifications.

3. Checking the Menu:

When you arrive at a restaurant, carefully review the menu. Look for keywords that indicate whether a dish might contain ingredients you need to avoid. Many menus nowadays include symbols or labels for gluten-free, dairy-free, or other special dietary options.

4. Asking Questions:

Don't hesitate to ask questions about menu items. If a dish isn't clearly labelled or described, ask your server for more information about its ingredients. You can inquire about potential allergens or ingredients that might trigger your psoriasis symptoms.

5. Modifying Dishes:

Many restaurants are willing to accommodate dietary requests and modifications. For example, you can ask for a sauce on the side, substitute certain ingredients, or request grilled instead of fried options. Just remember to make your requests politely and thank the staff for their assistance.

6. Bringing Your Dish:

If you're concerned about the available options, consider bringing a small dish or snack that fits your dietary needs. This can be particularly useful if you're attending a potluck-style gathering. Bringing something you can enjoy ensures that you won't feel left out.

7. Practicing Flexibility:

While sticking to your dietary plan is important, it's also essential to be flexible when necessary. If you're in a situation where there are limited choices, try to make the best choice available without feeling too stressed. One meal off your regular diet isn't likely to significantly impact your progress.

8. Seeking Support:

Connect with friends, family, or online communities that understand your dietary needs. Sharing experiences, tips, and strategies can provide emotional support and practical ideas for navigating social situations. You might even find others who have successfully managed similar situations.

9. Focus on the Company:

Remember that social events are about more than just the food. Focus on the company, conversation, and overall experience rather than fixating solely on what you're eating. Engaging in meaningful interactions can help distract from any dietary concerns.

57

9

Meal Planning and Preparation

trategies for Effective Meal Planning:

Defining Clear Objectives:

Before you start feast arranging, characterizing your goals is significant. Think about your dietary requirements, psoriasis the board systems, and individual inclinations. Is it true that you are expecting to diminish irritation, keep a specific calorie admission, or spotlight on unambiguous supplements? Defining clear objectives will assist with directing your feast decisions and guarantee that your arrangement lines up with your well-being targets.

Making Week by week Menus:

Arranging your feasts for the week ahead gives structure and lessens the pressure of choosing what to eat every day. While making your menu, ponder remembering different food sources rich in cell reinforcements, nutrients, and minerals that can uphold your skin's well-being and in general prosperity. Expect to integrate a blend of lean proteins, entire grains, sound fats, and a lot of products from the soil.

Brilliant Shopping for food:

Your feast plan is just viable assuming that you have the right fixings available. In the wake of concluding your week-after-week menu, make an itemized shopping list. Coordinate the rundown in light of the segments of your supermarket to smooth out your shopping experience and stay away from superfluous buys. Adhere to your rundown to forestall motivation purchasing and keep fixed on your psoriasis-accommodating eating routine.

Preparing Fixings:

Concentrate profoundly on preparing fixings ahead of time. Wash, slash, and piece out vegetables, marinate proteins, and cook grains like quinoa or earthy-coloured rice. Having these fixings all set will altogether chop down your feast planning time during occupied non-weekend days, making it more straightforward to adhere to your arrangement. Store prepared fixings in impenetrable holders in the fridge for simple access.

Assortment and Adaptability:

While arranging your feasts, go for the gold. Try different things with various recipes, cooking strategies, and fixings to keep things intriguing and stay away from dietary dreariness. Be that as it may, likewise be available to adaptability. Life can be flighty, so having reinforcement choices for quite a long time when your unique arrangement probably won't work out is significant.

Careful Distributing:

Consider segment sizes while arranging your feasts. Indulging can prompt uneasiness and influence your psoriasis on the board. Use segment rules and pay attention to your body's yearning and completion signs to guarantee you're eating the perfect sum for your requirements.

Adjusting for Extraordinary Events:

Consider any unique events, occasions, or parties while arranging your feasts. On the off chance that you realize you'll eat out or go to a festival, change your feast plan in like manner. Look into menus ahead of time and pick choices that line up with your dietary objectives.

Following and Reflection:

Track your dinner plans and how they affect you. Note any progressions in your psoriasis side effects or by and large prosperity. The following can assist you with distinguishing designs and figuring out which food varieties or dinner blends turn out best for you.

Benefits of Successful Feast Arranging:

Consistency: Dinner arranging guarantees you reliably follow your psoriasis-accommodating eating regimen, which can decidedly affect side effects across the board.

Time Reserve funds: Arranging and preparing ahead of time save time during occupied days and decrease the probability of falling back on undesirable comfort food sources.

Diminished Pressure: Understanding what you'll eat disposes of the pressure of going with last-minute choices, particularly when time is restricted.

Monetary Investment funds: By adhering to a shopping show, you can try not to purchase pointless things and decrease food squandering.

Batch Cooking and Freezing Meals for Convenience:

Batch cooking and freezing meals are valuable techniques that can significantly simplify your meal preparation process and ensure you always have nutritious options available, even when you're short on time or energy. These methods are particularly helpful when following a psoriasis-friendly diet, as they allow you to maintain control over your ingredients and avoid last-minute unhealthy choices.

Batch Cooking:

Batch cooking involves preparing larger quantities of certain dishes or components in advance. Here's how it works:

Choose Recipes: Select recipes that can be easily scaled up without sacrificing quality. Dishes like soups, stews, chilli, grains, and roasted vegetables are great candidates for batch cooking.

Preparation: Gather all the necessary ingredients and prepare them according to the recipe. This might involve chopping vegetables, marinating proteins, or pre-cooking grains.

Cooking: Prepare a larger batch of the dish than you would typically need for a single meal. Use a larger pot, pan, or baking sheet to accommodate the increased quantity.

Storage: Allow the extra batch to cool, then portion it into individual servings. Store the portions you won't be using immediately in airtight containers in the refrigerator.

Reheating: When you're ready to eat, simply reheat the pre-made batch. This minimizes the time and effort required for cooking, making it ideal for busy days.

Freezing Meals:

Freezing meals is a fantastic way to extend the shelf life of prepared dishes and ensure you always have a variety of options available:

Portioning: After preparing a meal or dish, portion it into individual servings. This makes it easier to defrost and reheat only what you need.

Cooling: Allow the portions to cool to room temperature before transferring them to the freezer. This helps prevent the formation of excess moisture that can lead to freezer burn.

Packaging: Use freezer-safe containers or bags to store the portions. Make sure to remove as much air as possible from the containers to prevent freezer burn.

Labelling: Clearly label each container with the name of the dish and the date it was prepared. This will help you keep track of how long each meal has been in the freezer.

Defrosting and Reheating: When you're ready to enjoy a frozen meal, move it to the refrigerator to defrost overnight. Reheat in the microwave, on the stovetop, or in the oven, depending on the dish.

Benefits of Batch Cooking and Freezing Meals:

Time Efficiency: Batch cooking allows you to prepare several meals at once, saving time during busy days.

Consistent Nutrition: By cooking in larger batches, you ensure that every meal contains the same balanced and healthy ingredients.

Reduced Stress: Knowing that you have pre-cooked meals available reduces the stress of last-minute meal preparation.

Avoiding Temptation: Having nutritious options readily available reduces the likelihood of reaching for unhealthy convenience foods.

Essential Kitchen Tools for Easy and Efficient Meal Preparation:

The kitchen tools you have at your disposal can significantly impact your cooking experience and the ease with which you can follow a psoriasis-friendly diet. Here's a closer look at some essential kitchen tools that will help you create delicious and nutritious meals while managing your psoriasis:

1. *Quality Knives:*

A set of sharp, high-quality knives is a fundamental cornerstone of any well-equipped kitchen. Different knives serve different purposes, such as a chef's knife for general cutting, a paring knife for intricate tasks, and a serrated knife for slicing bread. Sharp knives not only make cutting and chopping more precise but also minimize the effort required, making cooking a more enjoyable experience.

2. *Cutting Boards:*

Invest in a variety of cutting boards made from different materials (wood, bamboo, plastic) to use for various types of ingredients. This helps prevent cross-contamination, ensuring that bacteria from raw meats or other ingredients don't come into contact with ready-to-eat foods. Wooden cutting boards are a popular choice due to their durability and resistance to knife marks.

3. *Food Processor/Blender:*

These versatile appliances are invaluable for a psoriasis-friendly diet. A food processor can help you chop, dice, slice, and shred ingredients with speed and precision. Blenders are great for making smoothies, pureeing soups, and creating sauces. They enable you to incorporate nutrient-rich fruits, vegetables, and other ingredients into your meals effortlessly.

4. *Slow Cooker/Instant Pot:*

These appliances are busy cooks' best friends. A slow cooker allows you to prepare meals over a longer period with minimal hands-on effort. This is particularly useful for creating tender, flavorful stews, soups, and casseroles. An Instant Pot is a multi-functional electric pressure cooker that can dramatically speed up cooking times for dishes that traditionally require hours, such as grains, beans, and tough cuts of meat.

5. *Storage Containers:*

Having an array of storage containers is essential for keeping ingredients fresh and storing leftovers. Opt for airtight containers to prevent moisture and air from affecting the quality of your food. Glass containers are a popular choice as they are microwave-safe, durable, and don't retain odours or stains like plastic containers might.

6. *Meal Prep Containers:*

These containers are designed with portion control in mind. They are perfect for prepping and storing individual meals, making it easy to stick to appropriate portion sizes. Meal prep containers are also handy for taking your carefully planned meals on the go, whether to work, the gym, or while travelling.

7. *Grater and Zester:*

A grater is essential for quickly grating vegetables, cheese, or nuts for salads, sauces, and toppings. A zester is particularly handy for adding the zesty flavours of citrus fruits to your dishes without incorporating the bitter pith.

8. *Measuring Tools:*

Accurate measurements are crucial, especially when following specific dietary guidelines. Invest in measuring cups and spoons for both wet and dry ingredients to ensure your recipes turn out as intended.

10

Lifestyle Factors for Holistic Psoriasis Management

<u>**S**</u>**_tress Reduction Techniques and their Impact on Psoriasis_**

Symptoms:

Stress is a well-known trigger for psoriasis flare-ups and can exacerbate existing symptoms. The relationship between stress and psoriasis is complex, involving a cascade of physiological responses that can lead to inflammation and worsen skin lesions. This section delves deeper into the connection between stress and psoriasis, as well as various stress reduction techniques that can positively influence psoriasis symptoms.

Understanding the Stress-Psoriasis Connection:

When the body is under stress, it releases hormones like cortisol and adrenaline as part of the "fight or flight" response. These hormones can impact the immune system, leading to inflammation. In individuals with psoriasis, this inflammation can manifest as skin lesions and exacerbate existing flare-ups. Additionally, stress can affect the balance of neurotransmitters in the brain, potentially influencing itchiness and discomfort associated with psoriasis.

Stress Reduction Techniques:

Deep Breathing Exercises: Deep breathing techniques, such as diaphragmatic breathing or box breathing, can help activate the body's relaxation response. By focusing on controlled and deep inhalations and exhalations, individuals can reduce stress and promote a sense of calm.

Meditation and Mindfulness: Meditation involves focusing the mind on a specific object, thought, or activity to achieve mental clarity and relaxation. Mindfulness, a form of meditation, encourages being fully present in the moment without judgment. These practices can help redirect thoughts away from stressors and promote a sense of tranquillity.

Progressive Muscle Relaxation: This technique involves tensing and then relaxing different muscle groups in the body, promoting physical relaxation and easing tension. It can help individuals become more aware of their body's response to stress and learn to release muscle tension consciously.

Yoga and Stretching Routines: Yoga combines physical postures, breathing exercises, and meditation to promote relaxation and flexibility. Regular practice can reduce muscle tension, enhance body awareness, and contribute to stress reduction.

Art Therapy and Creative Expression: Engaging in creative activities like drawing, painting, or crafting can serve as a form of self-expression and a way to channel emotions. Creative pursuits have been shown to reduce stress and promote a sense of accomplishment.

Impact on Psoriasis Symptoms:

By incorporating these stress reduction techniques into daily life, individuals with psoriasis can experience several potential benefits:

Reduced Inflammation: Stress reduction techniques can help lower the production of stress-related hormones like cortisol, thereby reducing inflammation and the severity of psoriasis symptoms.

Improved Immune Function: Lower stress levels can support a more balanced immune response, potentially leading to fewer psoriasis flare-ups.

Enhanced Emotional Well-being: Stress reduction practices promote relaxation and emotional balance, which can positively impact mood and overall mental health.

Better Coping Mechanisms: Learning stress reduction techniques provide individuals with effective tools to manage stressors, helping them navigate the challenges of living with psoriasis.

Quality of Life Improvement: By managing stress, individuals can experience an improved quality of life with fewer disruptions from psoriasis symptoms.

The Role of Exercise in Managing Psoriasis

Physical activity has long been recognized as a cornerstone of a healthy lifestyle, and its benefits extend beyond just cardiovascular fitness and muscle strength. When it comes to managing psoriasis, regular exercise can play a significant role in improving both the physical and psychological aspects of the condition. Here's a deeper exploration of the role of exercise in managing psoriasis:

1. **Improved Circulation and Oxygenation:**

Engaging in regular exercise promotes better circulation throughout the body. Improved blood flow ensures that oxygen and essential nutrients reach the skin cells more efficiently. This enhanced oxygenation can contribute to skin health and support the healing process, potentially reducing the severity of psoriasis symptoms.

2. **Stress Reduction:**

Exercise triggers the release of endorphins, often referred to as "feel-good" hormones. These endorphins have a natural stress-reducing effect, helping to alleviate the emotional strain often associated with living with a chronic condition like psoriasis. Lower stress levels can lead to a decrease in stress-induced inflammation, which can trigger or exacerbate psoriasis flare-ups.

3. **Immune System Regulation:**

Physical activity can help regulate the immune system, which plays a central role in psoriasis. While an overactive immune response contributes to the inflammation seen in psoriasis, exercise can promote a balanced immune function. This balance may help prevent unnecessary immune system reactions that can contribute to psoriasis symptoms.

4. **Weight Management**:

Maintaining a healthy weight is important for psoriasis management. Excess body weight can increase inflammation and stress on the body, potentially worsening psoriasis symptoms. Regular exercise, combined with a balanced diet, can aid in weight management and contribute to healthier body composition.

5. **Psychological Benefits:**

Living with psoriasis can take a toll on mental well-being. Exercise offers psychological benefits by promoting a sense of accomplishment, improving self-esteem, and reducing symptoms of anxiety and depression. Engaging in physical activity can also serve as a positive distraction from the challenges of managing a chronic condition.

6. Immune Function Enhancement:

Moderate exercise has been shown to enhance immune function, promoting the production of immune cells that help combat infections and regulate inflammation. By supporting a well-functioning immune system, exercise can contribute to reducing the frequency and severity of psoriasis flare-ups.

7. Lifestyle Integration:

Incorporating exercise into one's daily routine encourages a more active lifestyle. This shift can have a positive domino effect on overall health, including cardiovascular fitness, joint mobility, and mental clarity. Adopting a more active lifestyle can contribute to better overall well-being and a more positive outlook on managing psoriasis.

8. Tips for Exercise and Psoriasis:

It's important to approach exercise with consideration for your individual needs and limitations. Here are some tips to keep in mind:

Start gradually: Begin with activities that are comfortable and gradually increase intensity over time.

Choose low-impact options: Psoriasis can affect the joints, so opt for activities that are gentle on your joints, such as swimming, walking, or cycling.

Stay hydrated: Proper hydration supports skin health and overall well-being.

Listen to your body: If you experience discomfort or pain during exercise, adjust your routine or consult a healthcare professional.

Incorporate flexibility and stretching: These can improve joint mobility and reduce muscle tension.

Maintaining a Positive Outlook and Focusing on Overall Well-being:

Living with psoriasis can be challenging not only physically but also emotionally. Maintaining a positive outlook and nurturing overall well-being is crucial for managing the impact of psoriasis on mental health, self-esteem, and quality of life. This section delves deeper into the importance of cultivating a positive mindset and offers strategies for fostering emotional resilience while dealing with psoriasis.

1. **Recognizing the Psychological Impact of Psoriasis:**

Psoriasis is more than just a skin condition; it can affect an individual's self-esteem, body image, and mental health. Acknowledging the emotional aspects of psoriasis is the first step towards addressing them. You are encouraged to reflect on their feelings and experiences, validating any negative emotions they may be facing.

2. **Setting Realistic Expectations**:

One of the keys to maintaining a positive outlook is setting achievable goals and expectations. Psoriasis may have periods of improvement and flare-ups. Encouraging you to set realistic expectations for your treatment journey helps prevent disappointment and frustration during challenging times.

3. Celebrating Small Victories:

Every step towards managing psoriasis is a victory. Whether it's a day without itching, a successful attempt at stress reduction, or finding a treatment that works, these achievements deserve celebration. Encouraging you to acknowledge and celebrate these small wins helps build a sense of accomplishment and motivation.

4. Cultivating Self-Acceptance and Self-Care:

Developing self-acceptance and practising self-care are essential for emotional well-being. You are guided through techniques to build self-acceptance by focusing on your strengths, fostering self-compassion, and reframing negative self-talk. Self-care practices, such as engaging in activities that bring joy, prioritizing relaxation, and nurturing hobbies, are also emphasized.

5. Seeking Social Support and Open Communication:

Psoriasis management can be made easier through social support. Encouraging you to open up to trusted friends, family members, or support groups about their experiences can alleviate feelings of isolation. Sharing challenges and successes with others who understand the journey can provide comfort and a sense of community.

6. Practicing Gratitude and Mindfulness:

Introducing gratitude practices and mindfulness techniques can help shift focus from psoriasis-related challenges to positive aspects of life. You can be guided through exercises such as keeping a gratitude journal, practising mindful breathing, and engaging in meditation. These practices foster resilience and improve emotional well-being.

7. Seeking Professional Help When Needed:

It's essential to recognize when the emotional impact of psoriasis is overwhelming. Encouraging you to seek the help of mental health professionals, such as therapists or counsellors, can provide tools to manage stress, anxiety, and depression effectively.